Darling CW

I think this

is just what

you and I

need — good

luck !

all my love

x x
x
Janice
x x
x
x x x

WHY GROW OLD?

VERNON LLOYD-JONES

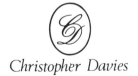

Christopher Davies

FIRST IMPRESSION 1980
SECOND IMPRESSION 1982
THIRD IMPRESSION 1986

Published by
Christopher Davies (Publishers) Ltd.,
P.O. Box 403, Sketty,
Swansea, SA2 9BE.

ISBN 0 7154 0554 3

*Printed in Wales by
Dynevor Printing Company,
Rawlings Road,
Llandybïe, Dyfed.*

DEDICATED TO

MY MOTHER

WHO WAS AGELESS

CONTENTS

AUTHOR'S FOREWORD

How many of us protest that 'age doesn't matter', when in the back of our minds we do care very much about the ageing process? Read any newspaper report and age is brought to our attention on every line e.g. 'Mrs Brown, aged 26, reported that her 5 year old dog and 12 year old son, had last been seen with their 72 year old grandmother.'

It is the purpose of this book to help you acquire an age-less appearance and approach to life. After all, if you care for your car, then you polish and protect the bodywork to enhance its appearance, whilst you pay similar attention to the unseen mechanical parts so that it will last longer. How much more important is your own body? Therefore, care for your external appearance and, more important, look after the machinery of your body — the internal organs.

In the following chapters I will give you an outline of how to retain your youthful appearance, as well as hints on how to maintain good physical condition. You have already taken the most important step in this direction by picking up this book — now for the action.

CHAPTER I

THE OLDER WOMAN STRIKES BACK!

'You're not getting older, you're getting better.' How can you believe this when for the last decade society has been on a youth kick that is unique in the world's history? Now it's time for you to strike back. You are not getting older, but better!

The purpose of this book is to prove that it is really true and to show you how to express this truth in the way you look and the way you feel. In the eyes of your friends, husbands and children you can change your image from a middle-aged woman to the figure of an ageless woman.

In 1900, the average life span of a woman was fifty so that at thirty women were middle-aged and could only expect to live another twenty years. Today the average woman can expect to live for seventy-five or eighty years and by the year 2000 a woman will expect to live to be one hundred. What, I wonder, will she do with this new lifetime? Not much, if she clings to the old fashioned idea about growing old gracefully, but plenty, if she is willing to smarten up (literally), sharpen up (fashionably) and join this modern era.

It's not as easy as it sounds but it's worth it. Every day I see women who come to me for help. As you might expect, depression is one of the first symptoms and many of the inexplicable depressions of the menopause can be traced to the apparent loss of sexual identity.

Uncertainty about her role as a mature woman is often reflected in unfeminine dress. She may feel as feminine as ever but thinks: 'At my age I don't want to make a fool of myself.' She wears a tailored suit, so-called sensible shoes and a short serviceable hair style. She's 'through with sex and all that nonsense' and this feeling of uncertainty is revealed inevitably in her physical appearance.

Fatigue and run-down condition go hand in hand with overweight and everyone knows what this does for morale. Convinced that she is no longer desirable, the middle-aged woman expresses this wan personality firstly in her body language and then eventually, her own negative attitude to herself is reflected in the attitude that other people have towards her. This results in a self-defeating vicious circle.

Is there an answer to her problems? Of course there is. She can become an *ageless* woman — neither old nor young. She can become aware of the power of mind over matter and adopt an attitude that will create agelessness whilst rejecting those attitudes that make age a reality.

The older woman must have confidence, a confidence that is expressed in many many ways. Among these is her refusal to accept society's old-fashioned attitude about mature women. She knows that she stops being a woman when she stops thinking of herself as a woman and so she must express her femininity in a thousand subtle ways. The way she moves, the way she dresses and the way she feels. We will soon be learning how she does this!

We all know of the famous legendary women whose faces are on the front pages of the fashion magazines and Sunday supplements but let me introduce you to some real women, women I have seen in my consulting rooms.

First, there's Jean. When she came to see me she was a rather dowdy, depressed matron. The youngest of her three children had just got married and her own marriage was breaking up. Today she is beautiful with the figure of a teenager and she does a part-time job with a cosmetic company. Still happily married her enthusiasm and outlook have changed her husband's life too. Indeed, when he looks at his wife it makes him feel younger!

Then there's Margaret who was 50 when she came to see me. She was immersed in her home-making, cooking, sewing and gardening and she had put on a lot of weight. She said to me, 'Oh well! at my age this happens. I'm not going to kill myself dieting and anyhow, my husband likes me the way I am.' I didn't see her then for about 18 months when she told me her 25 year marriage had suddenly fallen apart but, unlike some novels, this story has a happy ending. She is now 30 pounds lighter and has a new hair style. This, together with the correct use of makeup has turned her into a beautiful woman. But, it isn't fashion alone that turned her into a beautiful woman, her confidence and the way she carries herself have all combined to make her a fascinating woman and now there is a new man in her life. She has learned slowly and painfully but she has also learned well.

Now these two women had several things in common; they became determined to beat age; they were willing to try new ideas, new ways of thinking and to start on first things first. What does come first in this age game? Your physical appearance and that is what this book is dealing with in the first few chapters — 'the outer you'.

The sensible older woman will reject the idea that fashion

and beauty are frivolous; she will also reject the idea that makeup and new hair styles are only for the very young. The sensible older woman will also reject the idea that the body is just a thing to be covered up and fed. She will respect her body and her diet. She knows she can choose to be healthy and slim. She refuses to give up as so many women do; she will not spend her mature years trapped in a mass of weak, flabby flesh!

In this book I will try to describe a diet and exercise programme that can rapidly change you from middle-aged to ageless. It will tell you how to be healthy and well-adjusted, so that you can sail painlessly through those dreaded years of the menopause. Then there are the mental attitudes that are so important in fighting age. A lot of this book will deal with positive attitudes. What are they? How to develop them and what they can do for you. Now for some of these positive attitudes to start you on your way.

1.   Knowledge

You have taken an important step towards becoming ageless when you decide that your opinion is more important than that of your next door neighbour or indeed the old-fashioned opinion of society and have the courage to turn your back on yesterday and become the woman of today.

2.   Courage

You must have the courage to think you are not getting older but your potential must go beyond the goal of just being younger. You are getting better because the older woman can have the best of both worlds — maturity and youth. Use this knowledge for mental accounting.

Study your attitude toward yourself as a woman. Do not allow negative attitudes to develop. Do not become accustomed to thinking of yourself in limited terms — that is very bad. Instead, build up a positive attitude about yourself. This book will give you the foundation to build upon.

3. Never be Negative

Never say things like 'When I was young' or 'None of us are getting any younger' or 'I'm not as young as I used to be.' It has been said that when a word is spoken a chemical change takes place in your body and, because of this, the body may be renewed or transformed through the spoken word. Of course, the reverse is also true, so build yourself up.

4. Look at middle-aged women you know

If there are some middle-aged women who seem special to you, look at them, can you see what makes them special?

5. Now let's have some Real Action!

Come on let's get started!

CHAPTER II

DIET

If you are really determined to look younger you must realise that fat is old; with every pound overweight you add a year to your age. Don't believe that fat people are happy people. I have never met a happy 'fatty'. On the other hand, a slim well-proportioned figure helps you win the age game because it implies vitality and health. A slim, active body inspires love and admiration, a dumpy, flabby body is usually doomed for sitting down.

How many of you, after reading the last paragraph, are saying, 'Oh my God! I must lose two stone.' Those extra pounds loom like Mount Everest, a frightening, impossible challenge.

Now setting this impossible task does have its advantages. The thing is not to be discouraged and not to say to your friends, 'Of course fat runs in our family.' Actually, very few women need to lose more than a stone to change their image.

Naturally, to lose weight, you must make sacrifices; you will have to give up those big meals, those cream cakes and sweets and those extra cups of tea and glasses of sherry!

Mention the word 'Diet' to some people and it's the dreaded four letter word, the word that hovers like a cloud over every meal. Overweight is as much a symptom of malnutrition as underweight. This is the opinion of many doctors and nutritionists. Adele Davis, in one of her books, states: 'Much over eating may be an unconscious urge to obtain nutrients one's body needs, though most overweight persons eat far less than do their slender, energetic friends. To lose weight successfully, one must concentrate as never before, on obtaining nutrients which increase energy production.'* She adds that to be overweight not only can cause you to be a target for deficiency diseases, it can, itself, be a deficiency disease.

If you want to know how old your body is, pinch the skin on the back of your hand. The elasticity of your skin will tell you if you're older than your years. If your skin is elastic and snaps back it means that you are physiologically young. If the skin is flabby and the pinch mark just creeps back then you are creeping to old age.

Now that I have ruined your day, check out these other signs of age and see how you rate:-

1. Hair and nails break easily and lack lustre.
2. Facial expression is drawn and tired.
3. Muscles lack tone — particularly facial muscles and the back of the arms — breasts are flabby and tend to droop.
4. Eyes are puffy, ankles and hands tend to swell, especially in the mornings.

What was your score? Bad? I thought so. Well don't despair, every one of these ageing characteristics can be a common symptom of protein deficiency. If you are in good health, you can dramatically reverse these signs by supplying your body with all the protein it needs.

---

* Adele Davis, *Let's Get Well*. George Allen & Unwin, 1966.

Every child in school learns that protein is important in human nutrition; every weight-conscious woman has heard of the benefits of a high protein diet. True, everyone talks about protein. To reap the many benefits that can be derived from a protein rich diet, let's have a quick review.

1. Every cell in the body contains protein.
2. If the body's protein needs are unfilled, then the body feeds on the protein stored in the less important body tissues in order to rebuild essential organs.

How much do you need? How much are you getting? Nutritionists recommend 65 grams of protein each day for men and 55 grams for women but many would consider this too low to rebuild a body that's showing signs of deterioration. Some experts suggest that an easy way to figure your protein is to base the total day's requirements on half a gram for each pound of your ideal weight. Suppose you should weigh 120 pounds — simply divide by two and you know that 60 grams of protein is what you need.

Here is a short list of items high in protein:- Brewers Yeast, Wheat Germ, Soya Beans, Millet and Nuts.

At first glance the following menu plan may look like the usual high protein, low carbohydrate diet. Take another look and you will see some not so common foods mentioned.

Breakfast	**Protein Grams**
1 Orange	0
1 Egg scrambled with 1 teaspoon of Soya Oil	8
1 inch cube of cheese	8
1 slice of whole wheat toast	3
	19

OR

½ Grapefruit	0
½ cup of Millet with 1 Teaspoon of butter,	
sprinkle with 1 tablespoon of	
Wheat Germ	13
Sweeten with Honey	3
	——
	16

Mid-Morning

8 oz glass of Skimmed Milk	8
1 Tablespoon Soya Lecithin	0
	——
	8

Lunch

(This can be very light if you wish to
   lose weight).
A Green Salad with ½ cup cottage cheese,
   oil and vinegar dressing   20

OR

1 Portion cheese	12
Celery, Carrots & Lettuce (as much as you want)	
10 almonds	2
	——
	14

OR

½ cup Yoghurt & Fruit with ¼ cup of cottage cheese	15 ½

Dinner

4 ozs of Calf's Liver, grilled onions	23
½ cup Broccoli with 1 teaspoon of mayonnaise	2 ½
½ cup Yoghurt with Fruit & 1 teaspoon of honey	5 ½
	31

OR

½ cup (4 ozs canned Salmon)	17
½ cup green peas	2 ½
½ cup Beetroot	½
1 Apple	1
	21

EVERY DAY EAT:-

1 Piece of bread (Wholemeal or Rye)
1 Orange
2 Green Vegetables
3 Tablespoons of Vegetable Oil
1 or 2 teaspoons of Kelp
3 tablespoons of Lecithin

All milk should be skimmed milk. Drink 1 glass of water after every meal. Why? Water is necessary in the digestion of protein, and will help you process it effectively, and so prevent constipation.

There is some evidence that the 'fountain of youth' is indeed in your own kitchen. Many nutrionists believe that the body ages because its repair processes are no longer efficient. Whilst old age may manifest itself in a variety of degenerative conditions, each with its own symptoms, this degeneration stems from a single cause — the degeneration of individial cells and the body's inability to replace those cells.

If ageing is the deterioration of our cells then let's make them healthy again by providing those substances that nourish and repair them directly. The substance that fulfills this need is D.N.A.* — the body's master chemical for building new cells. It is to be found in:—

1. Fish (especially Sardines)
2. Peas, Lentils and Soya Beans
3. Liver
4. Beetroot
5. Spinach
6. Nuts

Lecithin

Too little is known about Lecithin (pronounced 'Less-i-thin'). It is found in every cell and organ of the body and some experts feel that it is essential for cell regeneration and may retard the ageing process. Lecithin is so important in weight control because it helps to re-distribute body fat. Perhaps this is because Lecithin is a fat emulsifier. In the

---

* Dioxyribonucleic acid

body Lecithin breaks down the fatty substance, Cholestrol. Lecithin contains the B Vitamin, Choline, which contributes to the health and strength of muscle tissue. Lecithin is available naturally in soya beans, but can be bought in any health shop in the form of tablets, powder, granules or capsules.

Kelp

We get Kelp from seaweed. It is a very popular new addition in reducing diets. Kelp is rich in iodine, the mineral that helps the Thyroid gland to function properly and produce the correct amount of the hormone called 'Thyroxin'. This hormone controls the speed of your life processes (or metabolism). It behaves much like the accelerator in your car. This is where Kelp comes in. This iodine-rich food can gently nudge sluggish Thyroid glands and stimulate them to produce the amount of Thyroxin your body needs. Since Kelp is a food and not a drug it can be safely added to anyone's diet. Many scientists say that Kelp contains all the elements needed for cell regeneration and repair. It is available from health shops in the form of tablets, powder or capsules.

Skin Care

If you eat what I call 'Beauty Fuel Food', your face will soon show how they work. All women need creams and lotions to cleanse and lubricate the skin on the outside. I'm going to give you a few inexpensive recipes. If you have a dry skin try the following.

You will need:-
1 Small Jar
1 Bottle of Wheat Germ Oil
1 Pint of Whipping Cream.

Mix the oil and cream together until it is quite thick and keep in a refrigerator. If you want to make this cream rich in vitamins you can add 2 capsules of Vitamin A 25,000 i.u. and 5 capsules of Vitamin E 200 i.u. Puncture the capsules with a pin and add to the above cream before whipping.

A Very Cheap & Marvellous Face Pack:-

2 Tablespoons of Acacia Honey
2 Tablespoons of Dried Milk

Mix together to a paste. Apply to face and neck, leave on face for approximately 15 minutes, wash off in warm water. Pat the face with a soft towel. You can use this face pack about once a week.

Lemon Refresher

½ Pint of distilled water
Juice of 1 Lemon
Strips of Lemon Peel

Strain the lemon juice and add to the water. Shake vigorously. Add the strips of lemon peel (to get the scent of Lemon) use this as a cleanser.

Now, having read so far, have you decided what sort of person you want to be as you grow older? Do you want to waddle through what should be your best years as an over-weight, self-indulgent woman or do you want to be smart, beautiful and ageless? If so, you will have to change your life style from self-indulgence to self-respect and enjoy the fun and dynamic kind of life during the bonus years that your own self-discipline will give you.

CHAPTER III

FASHION

New and exciting fashion is the quickest way of changing your image. Diet takes weeks, new hair styles take hours but you can change a dress in minutes and the way you dress is the one aspect of life where you have absolute control.

It is so often said 'Don't follow fashion'. I think a woman should follow fashion if she wishes to look younger and here are three reasons why:-

1. Wearing fashionable clothes tells everyone you are not living in the past.
2. Wearing today's fashion has a wonderful effect on you, it makes you take a look at yourself with new awareness.
3. Looking up to date makes you feel young and ageless.

Sounds good doesn't it, but what if you feel uncomfortable in today's fashion when you have passed forty? Well, you can give in or fight. If you decide to fight back, you will wear modern styles with confidence. It is simply a matter of understanding fashion. If you understand fashion you can wear anything with authority.

If you understand how the world of fashion works it will

help you; it works on two levels. The first level is that fashion is motivated by profit; the other level will be of more interest to you. Fashion is not meaningless, on the contrary, it is the visual essence of our civilization. Fashion reflects the society in which we live.

Fashion designers in London, Paris, New York and Rome have the knowledge and the ability to tell women what to wear. Does this sound terrible? I think not, because fashion reflects each era in fascinating ways.

I think of fashion designers as architects. For instance, the dome of a Mosque looks like a Turban. Talking of hats, they have been out of style in this country for some time, other than for functional purposes — such as rain hats and sun hats — but the truly feminine hat with the veils and flowers is now a thing of the past. So you can see fashion is something not to be taken lightly, instead, study fashion trends and make it part of your way of life.

The way to spot new fashion is:-

1.   Notice hem lines — up or down?
2.   Belts worn above or below the waistline?
3.   Sleeve shapes.
4.   Dresses flared or body clinging?

All these things indicate fashion trends. In the 1950's the mood was elegant and formal, today the mood is much more towards casual clothes.

Choosing Clothes to Suit your Figure

Waistline

If you have a short waist choose clothes that don't have a waistline at all and choose clothes of one colour. If you have a different colour top to the skirt, this will make you look shorter than ever. Choose waistbands or belts with care — if you must wear a waistband make sure it is narrow to make your waist look longer.

If you have a long waist choose styles with wide belts or waistbands. Always choose a straight belt as this will make your body look shorter. Avoid styles with dropped waistlines and choose shorter jackets as this will make short legs look longer. Show as much leg as fashion will allow as this will give the legs a longer look. Choose two tone colours as this will make your body look shorter.

Choose colours with great care. Avoid the baby pinks and blues. These very pale shades are for babies only.

Fashion and your Face

Often you will see an older woman smartly dressed with a youthful figure, then she turns around and you see she has committed a great fashion blunder. Her make-up is the same as it was twenty years ago. Nothing creates the illusion of age more than out-moded make-up, except of course a face with no make-up on. If fashion is the mature woman's good friend then make-up (used correctly) is her 'Fairy Godmother'. Yet so many women fail to make use of the miracles that modern make-up can do. How do I know this? Well I lecture almost every night to groups of women and I study the faces looking back at me and so many of them are so out of fashion with their make-up. I can always see lots of Katherine Hepburns with the 1950's eyebrows and lots of June Allysons with the well-scrubbed look but wait, there's worse, I even see some Bette Davis's with the tortured red lipstick look. Then, of course, there are the Marlon Brandos'. Well, how else can I describe the women with the outdoor look, with the short cropped greying hair and leathery skin? If this description sounds unkind I hope you will say, as others have said to me, 'Thanks I needed that.'

Every woman's face needs make-up, but it is a 'Must' for the mature woman and when I say make-up, I really mean the lot — foundation creams, blushers and eye-shadows. A lot of women will say, 'Oh, I like the natural look.' Do remember the natural look is lovely but only on young children.

Try a new make-up. Try it at home during the day when you are alone. Look through a recent fashion magazine. Look at the faces, compare your eyebrows to the ones in the picture, the nose, the eyes, the colouring. Now go on, experiment, it will be fun and worthwhile.

You will look younger if you have an even tone under the eyes and the nostril area. You will look older if you have dark shadows under the eyes or heavy make-up around the eye area. Shadows and circles under the eyes make you look tired and old but it is easy to disguise these with a shadow cover. Choose a light colour cream for under the eyes. You will look younger if you use a beige foundation as a base, you will also look younger if you use a bronze blusher and get the healthy look of youth. Eye-shadow should be light in colour and used in the fold of the eyelid which will make your eyes look brighter and larger.

Now if you wear glasses you can look sensational in them if you don't let your eyes disappear behind them, so wear enough make-up to accent your eyes. Let the glasses be part of your fashion.

Hair Styles

Remember long hair is fine on very young girls but an older woman needs a short neat style. In his book 'Complete

Book On Hair', Kenneth Battelle, whose clients included Jacqueline Onassis, explains that hair should be healthy: this is the time for beautiful, luxurious hair, shiny hair, healthy hair. You will look ageless in hairstyles that are drawn softly back from the face. Never wear the hair pulled severely back, this tends to pull the skin and make the face look flabby.

If the hair is worn short you must pay special attention to the neckline. The back of the neck is one of woman's most feminine features, it should always be graced with softness at the hairline with a wave or curl. Here again pick a model or actress whose face is similar to yours and imitate her. Don't laugh. It is really easy once you have tried it, choose someone in your age bracket or better still a little younger. And what, you may say, about being original? Almost everyone looks a bit like some fabulous person in the public eye. Everybody is a 'Type' so choose your model and copy.

You may find your double among the following list:-

Sophia Loren	(Forty Plus)
Jacqueline Onassis	(Fifty?)
Zsa-Zsa Gabor	(Who Knows)
Marlene Dietrich	(70 Plus)
Barbara Cartland	(70 Plus)

It is a list of some ageless beauties and of course there are many many more. Study their faces, what makes them ageless? I would say health, care and a great desire to stay young.

Now should you Colour your Hair?

Well, will it make you feel better? There is no doubt grey is a symbol of age. It is estimated that over fifty per-cent of females in Britain use some hair colourant, so why shouldn't you? A more inexpensive way to make a dramatic hair change is streaking. It gives an exaggerated colour change and yet has some relationship to your own colouring.

The important thing to remember is that any hair style that will destroy your feminine image will make you look older. So, to keep young looking, wear a soft hair style. With a soft hairline you will win your way ahead.

CHAPTER IV

FIT FOR ANYTHING

Diet alone won't correct your figure problems. Diet will give your body the nutrients it needs. Diet will help you lose fat but the muscles need exercise. Regular exercise will keep you firm, keep your body in proportion, healthy and young.

What does it mean to be Fit?

It means:-
Stamina
Energy
Enthusiasm
Endurance

When you are in tip-top condition you can laugh at the calendar. A person can be slim and still out of condition — being physically fit starts on the inside. If your lungs, heart and blood vessels are out of condition then those old type exercises will not make you physically fit by themselves, something else is needed. The daily dozen won't do it, paddling around in a swimming pool won't do it, neither will a walk after dinner. There is only one type of exercise that will bring you rejuvenating benefits and once you have tried it you will be sold on it.

Aerobics

Aerobics means living, acting or occurring only in the presence of oxygen which means simply that everyone of us is practising aerobics. We are all 'Aerobs'; it just means that some of us are more efficient than others in processing the oxygen we breathe. Oxygen is the key factor in turning the food we eat into energy. A well-developed oxygen processing system means that you burn fuel (your food) quickly and efficiently to produce energy. The main object of an Aerobic Exercise Programme is to increase the maximum amount of oxygen that the body can process within a given time. It is dependent on the ability to:

1.   Rapidly breathe large amounts of air.
2.   Forcefully deliver large volumes of blood throughout the body.
3.   Effectively deliver oxygen to all parts of the body.

In short, it depends upon efficient lungs, a powerful heart and a good vascular system.

However, through inactivity, the lungs, heart and blood vessels can become inefficient to the point that the slightest exertion leaves you huffing and puffing for air because your body needs more oxygen but the processing plant cannot deliver. The result is that the slightest exertion is unpleasant, produces fatigue and is religiously avoided.

Often during my lectures I hear people say 'I'm in tip-top condition, I run a home without help, I do all the shopping and play golf.' I have heard a thousand variations on this theme. Does it make sense? Test it yourself. When you are out shopping look at other women — how many do you see walking with a springy athletic stride and a lively expression? Most of them you see are trudging around with slumped shoulders, flabby thighs and drooping bosoms. Many of them look as if they are being held up by their shopping trolleys. In fact they are out of condition.

Research has proven that the conditioning effect takes place after about fifteen minutes of exercise. You must exercise until you begin to puff and then keep on exercising (and puffing) over a period of time. If you swim for a minute and then stop your body recovers from the slight demands made on it and you will not have accomplished any conditioning. This is why most programmes do not develop conditional fitness. You do an exercise, you start to puff a little, then you stop. Even the after-dinner walk will not do it, if you are walking at a pace that doesn't push your body to some degree.

As you gradually develop conditional fitness you will become healthier and have more energy. Once you are in condition exercise will not be tiring, it will become relaxing and stimulating and, a bonus for you, most figure problems will disappear.

To keep young you must exercise and the sooner you start the better you will become. It does more than get your figure into shape, it gets you into shape. Caution! One thing is certain, if you are not in condition you must not throw yourself into strenuous exercises but work up to it. Chances are you have spent twenty years getting out of shape so it is only fair to invest six months getting back into shape. Be sensible — you want to *become* fit, not *have* a fit.

How to get Started

Have a physical check-up. It is essential for two reasons:-

1. To find out if there is anything seriously wrong with

you. I would feel dreadful if you dropped dead with this book clutched in your hand.

2. When you have your doctor's assurance that you can undertake the exercise programme I am going to describe, you won't be frightened with a little puffing and accelerated heart beat or even a stitch in the side. Always remember it is the huffing and puffing that is good for you.

Now get Started

The safest and most beneficial exercise is to go outside and start walking but I don't mean a leisurely stroll. Walk at a brisk but comfortable pace then build up to twenty-five or thirty minutes without stopping. There are a few important points to note in order to make this walking time produce physical benefits. First, good body posture is absolutely essential. You cannot slouch along and expect your body to perform efficiently. The erect body posture has two benefits, it aids good breathing and it also helps you to develop this posture even during the times when you are not exercising. The best way to describe erect posture is 'walk proud'.

Second, breathing. Do not try to do anything fancy with your breathing, just breathe naturally but through the mouth as much as possible. This will help you to take in greater volume of air. Now as you begin to huff and puff a little encourage your body in this more vigorous breathing so as to give greater expansion to the lung cavity which will help you to take in more oxygen.

Arms

Try not to swing them too forcefully; just let them swing

as naturally as possible. They will automatically work to a correct rhythm with the movement of your legs and hips. As you move quicker your arms will move more quickly; this will happen naturally.

Feet

Here again, just move naturally. Some women tend to step onto to the ball of the foot, you should guard against this. You want your heel to touch the ground as the body weight passes over the whole foot. Now if this sounds complicated, the best way is to step down almost flat-footed.

I must mention that you should wear good, supportive shoes but not sandals or something similar; just sensible, comfortable shoes.

Jogging

When you are able to walk briskly and comfortably for about thirty minutes without stopping, then you can start jogging. Walk briskly for about twenty-five minutes, then jog for five, then walk slowly for five minutes (to cool off); then another day you can walk for five minutes and jog for five minutes or adapt to a pattern that is comfortable for you. The important thing is, don't set a distance, just set a time and enjoy it.

How often should you Walk or Jog

If you start on the walking programme it should be more frequent than the jogging programme — at least five days a week. A good way of doing this, especially when you are just starting is to walk on alternative days then as you get fitter, you will find that you will actually want to do more. Walking or jogging every day will not be too much for someone who is conditionally fit but remember the body will dictate to you a comfortable rate.

As far as the Jogging Programme is concerned, once you have worked up to a good jog, then you should jog four days a week at least. Most joggers run more often than this. If you will stick with it through the initial stages, you will find you will want to and be able to do more — it's fun and very rewarding.

This may sound very simple and easy, and you may think too easy to have any effect. But wait until you have actually tried it and I'm sure you will be surprised that this seemingly easy programme will appear strenuous at first. I have found many teenagers who are unable to jog for five minutes at the beginning but eventually they build themselves up until they can jog for thirty minutes — a goal you can set yourself. This is a realistic goal for healthy, mature women, though it may take six months to a year to reach it.

By yourself

I know a lot of women prefer to exercise in groups but I think it is better to set your own schedule because firstly, it is flexible so that you can fit it into your day (an advantage to women with full time jobs) and secondly, if you exercise independently you can easily make adjustments to any change of plans. Also you have unlimited freedom of choice over where you do your jogging; you are not always confined to the same room. The whole world is your track and pleasant surroundings help make jogging an enjoyable experience.

And what will your Neighbours say?

I know that when I first saw people jog, I used to think

'look at them' but jogging has become such an accepted part of the British scene that today you will hardly rate any attention at all other than glances of admiration and, yes, even envy. Of course I understand many women prefer the companionship and encouragement found in exercise groups. The all important thing is, whether alone or in groups, do it because it is well worth it.

What will it do for you?

It doesn't matter whether you work alone or in groups. If you stick with it, you will be sold on the Aerobic approach to exercise and to jogging in particular because of what it will do for you. Here are some of the benefits you can expect:-

1. You will have more energy because the Aerobic effect increases the efficiency of your circulatory system. When you get more oxygen, it stimulates muscle tissue and you will feel alive. You will want to do things where before you just felt like sitting around.

2. More than likely you will change your dress size within six months (from larger to smaller, naturally) or sometimes instead of an over-all weight loss, you may change your proportions by converting fat to springy muscle and be able to wear a style you couldn't wear before.

3. You will sleep better. Your Aerobic Programme releases tensions that may be keeping you awake.

4. You will find an improvement in your complexion; the improved circulation that will develop during an Aerobic Programme feeds the tissues. In addition the conscientious jogger works up a sweat and perspiration which is one way your body eliminates waste

toxins. Your own hard earned perspiration is your skin's best cleansing agent.

5.   You will tighten your tummy and build up your bust. Jogging flattens and firms the stomach and also has a definite effect on the contours of your bustline. Swinging your arms as you jog tends to build up the pectoral muscles that support the breasts.

Will all this exercise stimulate your appetite?

No, it does just the opposite, Aerobic exercise regulates the appetite because it improved your circulation, stimulates your metabolism and helps you burn all the food you eat. This together with your vitamin B diet stimulates your entire system and gets rid of those 'hunger pangs'. What is more, Aerobic exercise will teach you so much about your body.

Exercise and Diet

A sensible diet with exercise means that you will be burning 100 per-cent fat, leaving your body firm and slender. There is increasing evidence that regular exercise is absolutely essential to the mature woman. The benefits of an Aerobic Programme are measured not only in the present but also the future. In the present it can bring energy and a trim body. In the future it can assure you of the over-all health that is essential to agelessness.

Regular exercise is not only good for your bones; it is good for your brain too. I find people who do not get enough exercise very often suffer from nervous tension and often have no energy. In contrast people who are active and get plenty of exercise find their brains alert. They are usually very good conversationalists and bouncing with energy.

Reality

Knowledge and choices in fashion, make-up, and hair styling can create an illusion of agelessness and that is good but diet and exercise are essential to make agelessness a reality. Increasingly there is proof that building a level of conditioned fitness is one of the essential ingredients in combating premature ageing. The old adage 'What we don't use, we lose' is so true of the vitality of the human body. Diet and heredity play their parts but research indicates that inactivity and premature ageing go hand in hand.

So, if you wish to be ageless — then don't just sit there — make up your mind and do the Rejuvenating Exercise as part of your way of life. The sooner you get started, the better off you will be. Let your next birthday be dismissed due to insufficient evidence.

CHAPTER V

DON'T ACT YOUR AGE

There is one thing that will date you quicker than knowing the names of all three Beverley Sisters and that is 'moving old'. You can have the best figure in the world, be right up to date with fashion and make-up, but if you 'move old' you will look old. The thing that determines whether or not you create a winning image, will depend on the message you send through your body. Do you move young or old?

It is so important for you to understand this subtle body dimension, because the way you walk, sit, the way you move your hands, all telegraph obvious messages to those around you. I find it sad that so many older women belong to the dead message department. The way a woman walks tells me if she is 'old and tired'. the way she sits tells me if she is just a passive spectator. The way she moves her hands tells me if she is engrossed in fussy trifles. And, of course, those messages in turn create a predictable response.

Suppose for instance you are forty, fifty or sixty — why show it with every move you make? With knowledge and a little effort you can use your body awareness and young movements to help you become ageless.

Body awareness and young movements can be learned very quickly and easily and the rewards you will receive on both a visual and an emotional level are wonderful. As you learn to act younger and project a vital image, suddenly you are no longer acting, suddenly the role is you — you become younger. The great celebrities know all the secrets of body language, that is why so many famous women remain young indefinitely.

Now, how are you so far? Well you have taken a massive step forward if you are aware of the great importance of body movement. A depressing number of women don't even know about it.

When I talk about body movement, I don't mean walking about with a book on your head; that teaches artificial movement and has nothing to do with real life. You want to move young, not like a professional model. Every woman can learn the simple, natural movements that will enhance her beauty and concentrate on those movements that will project her image in positive ways. No woman would go for a job interview or to a party carrying a placard saying 'I'm nervous' or 'I'm getting old' yet by movements and gestures many women are silently 'shouting' those very messages.

Use positive body movements to project a confident feminine image which does so much for your ego. The image you project can mean the difference between success or failure. A woman's image can help her husband get promotion, it can also influence an employer at an interview. This is no exaggeration as I have listened to Personnel Officers responsible for employing people.

Old Movements
Patting your hair, clutching handkerchiefs, smoothing your skirt, straightening your gloves (a terrible give-away) fussing with your coat until it is 'just so,' all these fidgety,

nervous, meaningless gestures are the signs of a spinster-ish fussiness. Actresses use these aimless, fussy gestures when they are portraying an older fussy woman. Always remember 'busy hands are old hands'.

Hands are such a give-away to age — an older woman tends to clutch at things, her handbag, her escort or the arm of a chair.

Gloria Swanson used clutching hands very effectively in the movie classic *Sunset Boulevard*. Her beautiful hands became like claws clutching at the gowns she wore, clutching at her cigarette and in the final scene clutching at William Holden.Her hands in fact took over the film, expressing all the insecurity and possessiveness of a frightened old woman. The young woman holds things casually, even Steve McQueen! Her hands are relaxed, her fingers are relaxed and flexible and close together.

Carrying too many things is another give-away of age. The older woman has with her little parcels, tiny purses that in turn are put in larger purses and so on. All this activity is inclined to make her look flustered, harried and yes, old. When you go out don't take all your worldly goods with you. Instead, pare down, simplify. Travelling light is for those who look young and of course those who think young.

The crooked little finger is another age tip-off, also the lace handkerchief. There is nothing wrong with using a lovely large handkerchief to blow your nose if that pleases you, but using it to dab your forehead or your mouth gives the distinct impression of an old lady. Fanning yourself with a large handkerchief is worse, it makes one think of rocking chairs.

If it is a warm day and you are perspiring use a good modern tissue and wipe your brow with a no-nonsense gesture then, when you have finished with the tissue, throw it away — if possible. Do not put it in your sleeve or your neckline, or even in your pocket. It could ruin the line of your clothes.

Walk Young

How does the matron walk? Sit down for a few minutes in a shopping area and watch some walkers. The matron will place her feet flat on the ground as if they were made of cement. She doesn't roll her foot from heel to the ball of the toes which gives a springy walk. No, she just stumps along on those two slabs placing them far apart as she takes each step. The whole impression is one of solidity and weight.

Because she walks with her feet so far apart her body rolls from side to side which gives a rather aggressive, masculine effect — now if you imitate this walk in front of a mirror, you will see what it really looks like. Not attractive is it?

Sex Appeal

Every man will tell you that the way a woman walks is the basic quality for sex appeal. When women are older and have let themselves go, they waddle. Younger women swing along with those big shoulder bags, they swing their arms. Older women hang on to their purses and hold themselves stiff. Sex Appeal? I don't really know what it is but I can spot it a mile away just by how a woman walks.

Look at a stunning woman walking towards you, analyse her walk. First of all she moves freely — without any impression of stiffness. Her arms swing easily from her shoulders. Her walk is the perfect visual expression of the ancient law: 'youth is flexible, age is inflexible.' She uses her feet placing the heel down first, transferring the weight to the arch. No wonder she moves smoothly. Finally, you see she is walking with her feet pointed straight ahead and close together. It is not the artificial walk of a model but a natural smooth movement. Interesting isn't it? Now that she is close to you, you can see she is not so young as she appeared from a distance — but not old, that's right, you have guessed it — 'ageless'.

How to Stand

If you have some old magazines or newspapers at home, you will see that ladies used to stand with one toe forward, the back foot turned out at an angle — that was considered the correct way for a lady to stand but, somehow today that pose looks affected, stiff and matronly.

Today's attractive standing positions are more flexible. The important thing to remember in developing ageless standing positions is that the pose must create a graceful, female curve. Here are two standing poses you can try:-

1. Place your right foot to the side. Bend your right knee in towards your left knee. As you see when you try this, it is not the model's pose.
2. Place your right foot directly to the right about ten inches and straighten the right knee, you could also place the right foot ahead of, but to the left of the left foot.

Hands

I am going to suggest a few hand positions. You will make your overall appearance more attractive if:-

1. Your hands are not too busy.

2.   One hand in pocket (not both) but don't push the pocket forward.
3.   One hand on hip (never both).
4.   One hand hooked into your belt the other hand down at your side.

These are only a few suggestions. There are many other attractive hand movements. Look at models and you will notice one thing immediately; these glamorous women are never photographed clasping their hands together. Their hands are always apart and this creates a feeling of movement and energy.

Hands clasped together are associated with old age. Hands of children are never together unless a child is told to sit with her arms folded and this makes a five year old look like a matron and remember it will also make you look matronly.

Sitting

If standing and walking tells you a lot about age, sitting can be more revealing.

The older woman will approach a chair warily and sit with her back arched in the chair, the older woman usually sits with her ankles crossed and both feet flat on the floor. The younger woman will move confidently towards the chair because she has thought what she is going to do before she does it. She simply bends her knees and sits down. She slides back so that her hips are against the back of the chair. She sits with her legs together in a graceful position. Remember that crossing your legs is not good for your circulation.

Getting up out of a chair is another way of separating the

girls from the grannies. The older woman will try to get up while her hips are solidly settled in the chair or, worse, she may need help to get up which may be great for the gallant young men in the room but does nothing for the woman's morale. The younger or ageless woman, she's smart, she knows that to get out of a chair she must put her weight (hips, legs and feet) in effective alignment so, of course, she moves forward in one graceful movement.

You may say it isn't always that easy with low modern chairs and settees but, the theory is still the same — get your body and legs in as close alignment as possible and just stand up. There you are — easy isn't it?

Movement

When you are sitting, conversing with someone, you can use forward movement to indicate interest as well as ageless vitality — this gives the flattering impression of being interested in every word that is spoken. Forward movement is not a trick, it expresses participation. You can use forward movement in two stages. If you really want to impress, at first sit back and as the conversation progresses, move your head forward, then to show more interest, lean forward from the waist.

Obviously you can't use this forward movement all the time or you will look as though you are going to end up in someone's lap. Sitting back can also be alluring if it is done with style. Remember it is the matron who creates the solid impression because she sits stolidly and square. The younger ageless woman sits so that her body-line has curves, tucking one leg under or sitting curled up in the chair. The impression of being so relaxed. This lack of tension gives an aura of ease and femininity. I can now hear someone saying 'but surely this pose seems terribly affected?' Most women have a 'thing' about being affected. The trouble with this attitude is that somehow it always seems to pre-suppose that the 'real you' is the least attractive you. But, why should this be? Why not let the 'real you' be the best you? I think being totally natural is not a very good quality. I know a baby is natural but babies do many unattractive things quite naturally.

No-one is natural; let's face it, everyone is playing a role. If you want to see natural behaviour go to a large store when there is a sale on or visit a nursery. If you are lucky enough to escape from a sale in one piece you can reflect on all the social graces that make women attractive.

No, I am afraid a lot of women use this 'be natural' attitude to opt out and resist change, and why? Because change requires effort. When you say 'I don't want to change', what you are really saying is 'I can't be bothered to make the effort.'

Tension

Controlled breathing develops body awareness and releases tension. Not only does it help tension but actually creates a state of mind. We all know that emotions are easily read by the way we breathe. We know that short gasping breaths indicate we are under strain, be it anger, fear or uncertainty and, of course, the reverse is also true. If we practise calm, deep and even breathing under stress we project an attitude of peace. We can actually create more positive mental states. This is nothing new — actors practise deep breathing exercises to express calm and poise and also to indicate age. An older woman is apt to punctuate her conversation with sighs, her breathing is shallow and uneven which reveals more about her than she would tell her best friend. But a woman who wishes to remain ageless has learned how to breathe or she wouldn't be ageless.

Breathing

We can live for a time without food, days without water but we cannot do without breath for more than minutes. Yet few people realise the correct way to breathe. Here are a few tips:-

1. Sit up in a chair as straight as possible.
2. Start to breathe deeply inhaling through the nose. Retain the breath for a count of three.
3. Exhale slowly through the nostrils to a slow count of six.
4. Count three beats between breaths. Repeat a number of times.

Don't overdo it — the increased oxygen you are getting from this deep breathing may make you a little light-headed but this feeling will pass. The soothing effect of this exercise will convince you how good it is. It does work; ask any actor.

Personality

There are actresses who mesmerise audiences through the force of their personality. Now you may not have the desire to draw a crowd but it is nice to be able to attract people, interest them and fascinate them through personality projection. It is also nice to know that when you leave a party the other guests will know that some of the sparkle has gone out of the evening.

What is projection? It is a way of expressing your personality in terms of energy or life force. It is a means of communicating that goes far beyond words. Warmth, love and friendship can be expressed through projection. Projection comes from the heart. How often are such sayings heard; 'my heart goes out to you' or 'my heart leapt with joy.' Now in order to project personality and feelings — warmth, interest, love, compassion or whatever emotion you choose, you must project them from the heart. Does it work? Absolutely.

How does it work? There are many theories ranging from the mundane to explanations involving metaphysical laws and cosmic energy. In its simplest form, projection consists of consciously directing your own positive emotions towards other people but, at its most powerful form it projects an aura of cosmic magnetism around the person who practises it. Here are a few guidelines:-

To hold an audience when you are speaking, you want to project your personality. Your eyes can maintain that electric current of concentration but, the instant your mind wanders your eyes will wander. The moment you go away mentally the audience, whether it is a few friends or a dinner party, will know at once. Total concentration on the audience is embodied in the eyes. The instant your eyes wander it will be a dead give-away that your thoughts are elsewhere and you have lost them. When I speak of eye contact I do not mean a fixing star, effective eye contact establishes the concentrated interest of the audience.

Watch television actors and you can observe how they hold the eyes of the person they are talking to. But, just concentrating on your audience is not enough by itself, you must also acquire the ability to forget yourself — you must be a good listener. To be a good listener I believe there are three basic rules:-

1. *Concentration.* Totally engrossed in the speaker.
2. *Eye Contact.* Look at the person speaking but not a dull glassy stare.
3. *Facial Expression.* Keep your face alive, it reflects your interest in what the speaker is saying.

Using these techniques of concentration and eye contact which we have discussed will reveal a true personality that seems today to be increasingly rare.

CHAPTER VI

THE PAUSE

The menopause couldn't come at a worse time. It descends upon women at the advent of middle age, when they have enough problems already. The children are growing up, involved in their own problems and glandular discoveries. Also when women reach middle age, their parents are nearing the end of their lives and this sometimes forces them to make other difficult decisions. Do you place that loved one in a home or turn your own house into a convalescent home, creating even greater tensions?

There are tensions, believe me, because just as children are growing up and moving away, marriages are also undergoing a period of strain, with personal relationships in need of re-evaluation. Then just when you need him most, you find your husband begins to have problems of his own.

Just as nature slugs you with the physiological fact of menopause, with an exquisite sense of poor timing society loads many difficulties on to you. Women must often wrestle with all those domestic crises while plagued with sleeplessness, the hot flushes, leg cramps, headaches and heart palpitations. Then who can blame a woman when with all this going on, she suffers from anxiety and tends to burst into tears at inopportune moments.

So what does a woman do at a time like this? Some turn to the womens' magazines, and how do they help? Most of them will tell her go get involved in various activities; support political causes, immerse herself in community work or provide gourmet meals for the family. If she can't succeed in all those roles simultaneously then she's failed as a woman — and she can well do without such information at this time.

The problems of menopause may be far in your future but since it can occur any time between the ages of thirty eight and fifty five, you may already be involved, or it may only be around the corner. In any case I am sure you have heard a lot of old wives' tales to make you look forward to the 'change' with uncertainty and dread.

What does the Menopause hold for you?

According to the old wives' tales, the symptoms range from losing your mind to losing your libido. Most doctors are only a little more encouraging — 'A lot of women go through the menopause with no difficulty' — they say. This may be true for some women, but there are others who suffer from mild to severe depression, insomnia, headaches, fatigue and all sort of aches and pains. Well why you ask do some women have an easy time and some women a difficult time? I'm afraid too many of the medical profession answer this question resignedly — 'Nobody really knows.' You are expected to give up, endure it all and grow old gracefully.

Why settle for this?

Do you have to wait, watching the calendar, dreading the approach of the 'change' and wonder if you will be one of the lucky ones, one who will breeze through it, or if you are already involved in the menopause, do you have to endure stoically what should be some of the happiest years of your life?

No you do not! You can decide right now to be one of the lucky ones. Decide now to sail through the menopause with the minimum of difficulty, physical and psychological. You can decide to be one of those remarkable women who copes with her problems with clearheaded logic and leaves the imaginary problems to the imaginary theatricals. In short, you can be an absolute beauty as you quietly experience an uneventful 'change'.

I am sure by now you are thinking that he's going to give us a pep talk on meeting these crises with patience, will-power and fortitude. Not me, no pep talk, because the most maddening and humiliating thing about this whole process is the patronising attitude of too many people, including doctors, that your menopausal difficulties are 'an over active imagination'. That is just not true. Many women do have an awful time during the menopause and it certainly is not their imagination. Many a woman experiences severe physical problems and these can cause mental problems if she doesn't receive help.

The Two Levels of the Menopause

The menopause is complicated because it takes place on two levels — chronological and physical. As I have mentioned before in this book, the mature woman in our Society goes through an identity crisis at this time in her life — 'I'm not young, yet I'm not old — so what am I?' The menopause causes her to ask one more perplexing — yes even traumatic question — 'Am I still a woman?' At this difficult time in her life, a woman's very sexuality is threatened. These are the chronological stresses and of course they can cause anxiety and depression, what else would one expect them to cause? I have written this book to help women to understand, recognise and to overcome these chronological stresses.

Physical stresses also occur by the impact of the physiological changes of menopause — these physiological changes can express themselves in mental difficulties. Just at a time when a woman is under the impact of chronological stress, she is clouted again by chemical changes. What makes these two changes so devastating is that the chronological and physical symptoms are mixed up together in the minds of the women who are having the problems; their perplexed families and the doctor so often fail to help.

To recognise the dual nature of the menopausal symptoms is the first step to solving them, and these problems can almost always be solved, as you will see.

But can they be Solved?

At about this point, you may be thinking 'It's stupid to paint such a gloomy picture, when one can supplement with hormones and they will take care of the menopausal problems.'

But do hormones really solve all those mysterious physical problems that are common during the menopause? Now it is true that hormone therapy may help. If so, count your blessings. You are one of the lucky ones. But there is a fifty-fifty chance that hormone therapy will cause more problems than they solve. Many women find that some common menopausal symptoms may be cleared up after supplemental oestrogen, but several other vague and apparently undiagnosable symptoms often take their place.

The fact is that some women can't tolerate hormone therapy for one reason or another, and if they cannot tolerate it no other treatment is offered beyond the inevitable sedatives and tranquilizers.

As the physical symptoms increase and the glandular stresses multiply the woman in menopause may very well develop problems with nerves. Remember that psychiatric treatment can no more help her physical problems than it can a broken leg. These very physical problems can only be corrected by physical means.

Let us look at Oestrogen Therapy

Many of the symptoms I have been describing have been attributed to the reaction of the body due to the waning output of oestrogen by the ovaries. Hardly one week goes by that doesn't see a newspaper story extolling the miracles of oestrogen therapy. Some of the conditions that oestrogen therapy can help are — hot flushes, depression, anxiety and insomnia. Some physicians estimate that oestrogen therapy gives marked relief to fifty per cent of their patients going through the menopause. But what about the other fifty per cent?

There are women whose past medical history makes the use of oestrogen dangerous. Any woman with gall bladder trouble should think twice before taking oestrogen. Recent studies indicate that post-menopausal women taking oestrogen are two and a half times more likely to have gall bladder problems than those not taking oestrogen.

Suppose you are one of the women whose medical history precludes the use of hormones? Or suppose your doctor has prescribed hormone therapy with disappointing results, and hormones are not the answer.

What is a woman to do?

In the past, women were expected to put up with all these discomforts, but not so today. Whether or not hormone therapy has made a contribution to every woman's life, it has brought a more realistic attitude towards the menopause, taking it out of the realm of whispered old wives' tales of odd behaviour and mysterious malaches. Now let us look at the problems of menopause and see them for what they are.

The medical profession has concentrated on hormonal deficiency but there is a new approach to the deficiency theory that is now gaining momentum. Most menopausal symptoms can be traced to nutritional deficiencies and these can be corrected as easily as you eat your dinner. The women who are placed on a proper diet supplemented with Vitamin B.6 and Zinc will sail right through the menopause without difficulty.

Stress

Poor eating habits cause nutritional deficiencies, but nutritional deficiencies can also be caused by stress and the menopause years are filled with stress. There is the physical stress caused by the hormonal changes; mental stress because during the menopause years, a woman has to make important decisions — about her growing children, her family and her marriage. Then there is chronological stress when one must re-evaluate one's role as a woman. These stresses magnify one with the other. According to Adele

Davis 'When menopause symptoms are severe, the condition should be looked upon as another form of stress'.

Stress increases the body's need for all nutrients and the problems at menopause are caused by a diet deficient in the many nutrients required to meet the body's needs at this time. After all, when all nutritional needs are met, a healthy woman is unaware of disturbances. Prolonged periods of stress cause many destructive changes in the body. The first victims of prolonged stress will be the adrenal glands; their condition has a special relationship to the 'change'.

Let's get back to hormones for a minute. Do you know that you have a second source of oestrogen? As the hormonol output of your ovaries gradually slow down, the adrenal glands step up their production of oestrogen, and this can help the body to adjust gradually to the changes that take place during the menopause. This may well explain why some women have a difficult time and some don't. If your adrenal glands are exhausted because of mental and physical stress, they cannot produce the buffer of oestrogen that you desperately need — natural oestrogen. The result is that your body is not getting the female hormones it needs to function efficiently and all sorts of problems arise.

So how can you relieve the stress on the adrenals and keep them in shape to produce that extra oestrogen? The first thing is to remember that stress, no matter what the cause, stimulates the adrenal glands into action. At the onset of stress, the pituitary glands secretes two hormones that dash through the blood stream; proteins are broken down to form sugar for quick energy, blood pressure increases, the blood sugar soars and many many other changes occur.

A woman who is under continued stress is constantly rousing her adrenal glands into action. Unless steps are taken to protect these glands, they can become exhausted so it is easier if I explain to you how not to treat these over-worked glands.

Food and the Adrenal Glands

The first abuse of the adrenal glands usually starts first thing in the morning. You get up feeling terrible, not quite awake, not feeling hungry, so what do you do? Ah yes! the first cup of coffee; it tastes good and makes you feel better. The caffeine in the coffee gives a swift kick to your adrenals, forcing an alarm throughout your body and raising your blood level. You feel so good, so full of energy, that you're not even hungry so, of course, you miss the nutrients that your body really needs. Then comes the inevitable let-down. By ten o'clock you begin to feel droopy again; Ah yes! another cup of coffee or tea, so the caffeine and sugar deliver another kick to those already overworked adrenals. This is one of many ways you can keep your adrenal glands exhausted and unable to cope with the demands made on them. They are always too worn out to make the oestrogen that you need after forty.

How can you relieve the stress on your adrenals? Follow these simple suggestions:-

1. Follow the Super B Diet, for several reasons. First a high protein diet is essential to offset the demand on stress. Adele Davis in her book *Let's Get Well** wrote, 'During a single day of severe stress, the urinary loss of nitrogen has shown that the amount

---

* Adele Davis, *Let's Get Well*. George Allen & Unwin, 1966.

of body protein destroyed equals that supplied by 4 quarts of milk. Yet if such a tremendous quantity of protein can be eaten during that day, the tissues are unharmed'. Although your diet may not give you this much protein daily, it is certain that high levels of protein (that with Vitamin B) are advisable during the stressing menopause and pre-menopause years. And, speaking of Vitamin B, remember those wonderful foods — liver, wheat germ and yeast — they contain vitamin-like substances which are called anti-stress factors. Although much needs to be discovered about these nutritional elements, what is known is this: they have a fantastic ability to help the body withstand stress. Another anti-stress factor is found in green vegetables, so eat spinach, broccoli and lettuce.

There is a second reason for eating these fuel foods. They contain an element that is directly related to the condition of your adrenals — pantothenic acid, one of the B Vitamins. The richest natural sources of this vitamin are in liver, yeast, wheat germ, soya beans and kidneys. In addition vegetable oils are also essential to the healthy functioning of your adrenals. The unsaturated fats present in these oils contain an element called linoleic acid. A deficiency in linoleic acid causes a degeneration of the adrenal cortex and limits the production of adrenal hormones. In laboratory tests, rats that were lacking linoleic acid, and therefore suffering from impaired adrenal function, increased their production of adrenal hormones by 90 per cent when oils containing linoleic acid were added to their diet. The mixture of peanut, safflower and soya oils that I mentioned previously is an especially healthful combination that will give you the essential fatty acids you need.

2. Avoid sweets (you may not like this) but the unpleasant fact remains that sweets help to exhaust your adrenal glands. Sweets may be pleasant tasting but you must decide whether the consequences are worth it. When you find yourself drawn to that box of chocolates, think. Many authorities feel that the women who have a difficult menopause are the women whose adrenal glands are exhausted.

I cannot over-emphasize the importance of a proper diet especially the strict elimination of the rapidly absorbed carbohydrates in order to avoid the sudden rise in blood sugar. You may feel that you do not want to avoid these foods completely, it's certainly a good idea to go very easy on chocolate, sweets, cakes, and remember that soft drinks are high in sugar content.

No Coffee

You may by now be thinking of me as an old kill-joy but the case against coffee is so astonishing and so important to your well-being that we must face up to it.

Most people are sensitive to the stimulating effects of coffee. How often have you heard people say 'No coffee for me, or I won't sleep tonight' and limiting your caffeine intake to two or three cups of coffee a day won't take the sting out of this superstimulating chemical that we all drink so casually. Keeping you awake is one of the least damaging things that caffeine does. As I mentioned before, caffeine drinks beat those tired adrenals and stimulate them to further action. These poor glands then give you a momentary lift, but it is a lift that will let you down because the result will eventually be exhausted adrenals.

The effects of too much caffeine can be even more serious, it can bring on all the symptoms of an anxiety state. Other symptoms can be an irregular heart beat, irritability and drop in blood pressure. Coffee is the worst caffeine villain — but that meek cup of tea so famous for its comforting qualities will also give your system a good jolt of the old caffeine.

By now you are saying 'Oh! I can't give up tea and coffee.' Well here's the good news — you don't have to, you can buy decaffeinated coffee, which will taste like your old coffee but without the dangerous caffeine and also the tea without caffeine — these you can buy at any health shop.

Nutritional Deficiencies

Although your adrenal glands are often the first casualties in this battle against stress, specific nutritional deficiencies can be another result of stress.

Calcium

The most widespread nutritional deficiency among women in their forties and fifties is calcium deficiency. I see many women every day in my consulting room who are on the 'change'. I saw one woman recently who was upsetting her family with her quick temper and irritability and, to add to the confusion, she just as quickly and unexpectedly would turn an impossible tirade into a flood of tears. It was a mystery to her and her family but really the answer was

simple. Irritability, depression, headaches and hot flushes
— those typical menopausal symptoms that this lady was
suffering — were caused through calcium deficiency. Many
women have found that taking enough calcium to meet the
body's increased needs during menopause can overcome
those apparently mysterious menopausal symptoms in
record time — sometimes even in one day. In fact this one
patient I have mentioned came back to see me and to use her
own words she said, 'There's a miraculous transformation.'

The Nerve Mineral

Calcium is the element in the body which aids in the
transportation of nerve impulses. If the body is under-
supplied with calcium, the nerves become tense and you
become irritable. This, of course, causes stress. It is a vicious
circle. Another stress resulting from calcium deficiency is
water retention. When the body is under-supplied with
calcium, salt and water are retained and contribute to all
those unpleasant symptoms of pre-menstrual tension, a
condition that many menopausal women seem to
experience even though they are no longer menstruating.
You know the symptoms I mean — suddenly you put on
weight, you get headaches and become irritable. You can
correct this by a greater intake of calcium. I feel that 1.200
milligrams of calcium daily is essential for adults. Adele
Davis suggested even 2 grams daily.

The most convenient source is milk, one quart of
skimmed milk with one half cup of powdered milk will do
the trick but, of course, a lot of women wouldn't like this
form so I suggest tablet form.

My next chapter is Vitamins and how they will help you.

CHAPTER VII

VITAMINS AND MINERALS

Let me start this chapter by discussing the B Vitamins. In many experimental situations, mild deficiencies in any of the following B Vitamins have produced the following symptoms in dozens of both men and women volunteers:-

1. Vitamin B1 deficiencies result in:-
   Depression
   Fatigue
   Anxiety
   Quarrelsomeness
   Restlessness
   Lack of co-operation.
   Some suffered from insomnia, nervousness, sensitivity to noise and even hypochondria.
2. Pantothenic Acid deficiencies caused:-
   Irritability
   Depression
   Some volunteers became hot tempered and easily upset over the most trivial things.
3. Niacin deficiencies can cause these disturbing mental conditions:-
   Suspicions
   Depression

Imaginary Unfairness
Irritability

4. Biotin, another member of the B Complex family, is definitely related to mental equilibrium. A deficiency in biotin can cause mental depression which can develop in intensity and become panic.

These symptoms might well describe the mental state of many women who seem to change from normal, well adjusted individuals, to negative neurotics during middle age. The very important point to remember is this: many times these mental conditions develop even though a woman's life situation is happy and stable and in many instances her only problem is malnutrition and this can be quickly put right if you know how. I have seen many examples in my work and personal life but I think a friend of mine's experience is one of the most astonishing I have known ...

I had known Mary, a school teacher, for years. She had always been a placid person, but like all of us she had her every-day problems, but no matter what the crisis, she would always bounce back. About two years ago she developed a skin complaint, she had seen a Dermatologist and was taking antibiotics and thought it would soon clear up, but it didn't. A few weeks went by and I saw her again, her skin problem was worse and she was very depressed and told me that waves of panic came over her and that her husband Philip was very worried about her, she said that she thought she might be going crazy. I assured her she wasn't and had a long talk with her, then I mentioned diet. I found out that she was suffering from a severe deficiency of the B Vitamin Biotin. Her diet had been inadequate for years. She was just starting the menopause, which we have seen can cause stress throughout the system and increase the body's needs for nutrients.

I put her on a diet (rich in yeast, which is the best source of Biotin) together with Vitamin Supplements and a little rest. Mary was her former self again within weeks and those frightening and disturbing symptoms have never recurred.

Wonderful Vitamin E

More Vitamin E is found in the body than any other Vitamin. Every cell needs its full supply to function in top performance. There is a large concentration of Vitamin E in the pituitary, adrenal and sex glands. I am constantly being asked by people, if Vitamin E is an aphrodisiac.

So let's get the facts straight. Vitamin E is not an aphrodisiac, since the libido is a mental rather than a physical quality. But, numerous studies do indicate that Vitamin E is necessary for the health and vitality of sex glands. What Vitamin E does is to maintain the youthful function of these glands. In other words, Vitamin E helps things so that when the spirit is willing the flesh is not weak. So, it is a very friendly Vitamin in that respect.

More about E

According to the World Conference on Vitamin E a woman's need for Vitamin E increases ten-fold during her forties and if oestrogen is given, the need for E increases still further. Vitamin E stimulates the body's hormone activity and some physicians (those who are nutritionally orientated) even prescribe E instead of supplemental oestrogen and with very successful results.

Another annoying problem during middle age (and indeed often before) is the appearance of brown pigment

spots on the back of the hands, or on the face and sometimes around the edge of the hairline or the neck. These
'age' marks are just one more piece of the deficiency puzzle.

Research has shown that this pigmentation is the result
of a Vitamin E deficiency. It is not surprising then that these
pigment spots occur during middle age since the need for
Vitamin E skyrockets at this time. I am certain that there is a
dramatic increase in the need for Vitamin E when taking
hormones for any reason. In many lectures I give, I can very
often pick girls out who are taking the pill by the dark
pigmentation on their faces and necks. The significant
point is that these spots, formerly associated with age, are
now becoming common in girls in their teens and women of
all ages. Strangely, many of them develop this dark pigmentation on the upper lip.

The Age Fighter

A tremendous amount of research has been done on
Vitamin E. Dr Hans Selye (an expert on stress) has been
producing premature old age in laboratory rats by exposing
them to various stresses (noise, pollution etc.) and feeding
them on a diet deficient in Vitamin E. When he gave large
amounts of Vitamin E he found that premature aging did
not take place.

In fact, there is a lot of evidence to indicate that a Vitamin
E deficiency is a factor in bringing about a premature menopause. What is more, those who are in menopause and who
do not get increased Vitamin E appear to age rapidly.

Middle Age Spread

No-one really knows why a woman's body goes through
this fat distribution at middle age but it is a fact that many

women find their hips, arms, thighs and especially waists tend to fill out and this is not related to waning oestrogen output because, after all, middle age spread is common in men too.

Adele Davis said, 'I suspect that middle-aged spread of men is not so much the result of age or even too many calories, as of an undersupply of hormones caused by cumulative multiple deficiencies, of which Vitamin E is one.' She recommended 100 units of this vitamin, after each meal, for women whose weight was correct but whose 'faces were too thin and hips too large.' She said 'Though Vitamin E may not have done the trick, the weight of most of these women has been re-distributed' which was all they or I care about it.

Minerals

What is a mineral? A mineral is literally 'mined from the earth' and consists of a metal combined with some other group such as carbonate sulphate, oxide etc. which produces a stable salt, for example, iron sulphate. However, in the body the metals are not combined in this way but are complexed with natural body constituents such as hormones, proteins, enzymes and amino acids. When we talk about minerals in the body, we are referring to organic complexes of metals such as iron, calcium, zinc etc. or of non-metals like iodine as far as the functions of the body are concerned.

Minerals are as important as vitamins in maintaining the body in a healthy state. The body does not manufacture minerals and relies entirely on outside sources such as foods, supplements, inhalation and absorption through the skin, to ensure an adequate supply.

Iron

Iron is an essential component of haemoglobin, the pigment that gives the red colour to blood. Lack of iron means less haemoglobin in the blood and thus a reduced amount of oxygen is being carried around the body. Iron is an essential mineral that allows muscles to use this oxygen effectively, so it is not surprising that lack of iron leads to tiredness, apathy and breathlessness.

Magnesium

Magnesium exerts its action through the nerves. A nerve is normally surrounded by calcium and magnesium. When a nerve is stimulated these minerals are replaced by sodium and potassium. When the nerve returns to rest, calcium and magnesium move back to surround it. If there is magnesium deficiency, this is not possible so the nerve stays in a state of excitement. Thus it is not surprising that lack of magnesium leads to mental confusion and depression. People with nervous troubles often suffer from lack of magnesium. Magnesium controls the processes that replace old and worn out cells.

Two factors that contribute to magnesium deficiency are white sugar in the diet and stress. Magnesium is a natural tranquiliser. During the last half-century magnesium intakes have fallen, whereas dietary contents of fat, sugar and calcium have risen. High intakes of these foods and of Vitamin D* increase the need for magnesium. In the absence of extra magnesium they increase susceptibility to magnesium deficiency. An increased magnesium intake protects against heart muscle disease. Balance studies have

* Vitamin D is formed in the skin oils by summer sunshine, and the only other rich sources of natural vitamin D are in fish oils, particularly halibut and cod liver oil.

shown that the average Western diet is deficient in magnesium.

I spoke quite recently to a leading psychiatrist and he was convinced that more and more people were suffering from nervous conditions because of the lack of magnesium in the body caused by the eating of refined foods such as white sugar, white flour and frozen foods.

Zinc

Current research is establishing the importance of zinc in nutrition, and bringing to light evidence of deficiency in a wider range of the population than was originally thought.

Zinc functions as a constituent of the hormone insulin, which controls blood sugar levels. High levels of zinc are found in the prostate and in the reproductive organs of both sexes. It is involved in every stage of the female reproductive process. Zinc has been found to function in the prevention of prostate trouble, preventing the hardening of the arteries. A lack of zinc can give rise to skin diseases. Many diseases and drugs cause lowering of body zinc levels, in particular, women on the pill are prone to deficiency.

Ginseng

Every lecture I give and every talk I give on radio I am always asked 'What is ginseng?' and I really go to town on this one. I, myself, take ginseng every day. You don't have to. It's not a drug and it is not habit forming, but I feel so wonderfully well since I've been taking ginseng that I will always take it.

Well what is ginseng? It is a herb, a root grown in Korea and several other countries. It is comparatively new to this country, but the Koreans and Chinese have used ginseng for over five thousand years. Since the very first time it was prescribed to a patient millions of prescriptions containing ginseng have been dispensed and in fact, are listed in ancient writing by many practitioners. It is still a major medicament in both China and Korea.

The Wonder of Ginseng

Ginseng takes about six years to grow and when the root is taken out of the ground, nothing will grow in that part of the soil for a few years because it takes every mineral out of the ground.

Ginseng as Panacea

Ginseng has been prescribed for treatment of many illnesses. G. A. Stuart tells us that in China, ginseng has been considered helpful in stress conditions and fevers of all kinds. In China it is part of the army's medical kit.

Astronauts were given ginseng to fight mental stress. In a recent BBC interview I gave, I mentioned that the athletes who went to the 1976 Olympic games were given ginseng, the interviewer corrected me and said only the Russian athletes were given it. My answer was 'Yes, and they had the most gold medals.' Many many claims have been made about ginsent. I myself have seen some remarkable results. Not one day goes by without my seeing patients who feel so much better since taking ginseng.

I know at the lectures I give someone always asks in a whisper, 'Is it an aphrodisiac?' My answer to that is 'Sportsmen take it to play better, a lot of people doing Karate take it because it quickens the reaction. So if you feel better you do everything better'.

A tremendous amount of research has been done with

ginseng and is still continuing. Analysis so far has proved that ginseng contains many beneficial organic acids including:—

Citric
Ascorbic
Fumaric
Isocitric
Linollic
Oleic
Tartaric

It also contains a number of amino acids and the minerals Iron, Copper and Cobalt are just three of a very wide range of minerals to be found in ginseng. Vitamins found in ginseng are Vitamin B.12, Biotin, Thiamine and Riboflavine.

I could go on and on singing the praises of ginseng. Many books have been written on this subject and I felt I had to mention ginseng in this book.

CHAPTER VIII

WHAT HAS HAPPENED TO YOUR MARRIAGE?

Nothing, after twenty or thirty years of marriage, is a very common answer. But, if you think nothing has been happening to your marriage, you are wrong because next to that crisis time known as the 'Seven Year Itch', the middle years of a marriage are its most vulnerable, that is the time when the relationship is usually put away in moth balls or is cancelled due to the lack of interest. In other words at a time of life when both of you are facing all the physical and emotional changes brought on by the advent of middle age, your marriage is going through a radical change too.

But, with a little knowledge, some effort and a great deal of wisdom, not forgetting the dash of humour, you can help your marriage change for the better.

Just what is it that ails the middle-aged marriage? Someone once said 'Marriage must conquer the monster that devours, its name is Habit' and that monster *habit* seems most at home in the bedroom. My advice on this one is don't be intimidated by sex manuals, use your own imaginations.

Here is a simple test that will tell you more about your relationship than any marriage counsellor. Go out alone with your husband and have dinner, you may have done this often before but this time pay close attention to the subjects of your conversation. What do you have to say to each other? Is your conversation totally about domestic trivia? When should we decorate the lounge? The garden needs doing. What about the winter sales? A discussion about your insurance policies. Test yourself and you will be appalled by such trivia. One person I asked to do this test came back to see me and she said 'You are right, we are boring each other to death.'

Well I don't think there is any excuse for being bored in life and I will be discussing several techniques that will help you to put some sparkle back into your marriage. But let's continue with our analysis for a moment.

Memories

Do you find that our dinner-table conversation is almost solely devoted to memories? If the theme of your time together is strictly a rememberance of things past, your relationship is surely floundering in the dangerous realms of marriage boredom. If looking back is all you have in common, then you are in trouble.

I am not against memories, on the contrary I believe that memory is one of the miracles of the human mind, but nostalgia, like perfume, should not be over-done. In fact, memories should play a relatively small part in your life and often memories don't mean the same things to two people. For example, a wife may look back to carefree times when the children were young, when they lived in a small house and life was simpler. But, to the husband, those early years may bring back unpleasant thought of when he was starting his career, his frustrations and even uncomfortable pictures of the man he used to be and would rather forget. He doesn't want to be reminded of the early years and he won't thank you for constantly pulling him back to an unhappy time.

Or, maybe he is the one who is always looking back with the bitter-sweet conviction that things will never be as satisfying as 'the good old days'. If so, then he needs your help. Blast him out of that rut. Remember that if memories play too large a part in your life together, it reveals that the present and future are not meaningful and that you and your relationship are not growing. You have allowed your present and future to become so drab that you have to escape to the past and more than likely to a romanticised version of the past that is more pleasant in memory than it ever was in actuality. So, whatever your age, be very wary of over-indulgence in memory trips, they are very bad medicine for the ailing middle-aged marriage.

Communication

Rebuilding those lines of communication can bring new and exhilerating levels of intimacy to your marriage relationship. 'Getting to Know You' should be the theme song for your next evening out together and a good way to start is to listen. Encourage him to talk. Do you find that difficult? If that is the case, then you have learned a lot about your relationship already. Now with a little effort you can draw him out, and you will inevitably be surprised at what has been simmering in his mind.

You really will be quite shocked as to what is actually going on in his head. You may think you know all about his job, his hobbies and his hang-ups but how does he really feel about his job? What is the satisfaction that he gets from his hobbies? And, why the hang-ups?

How much does he know about what has been going on in your head? Have you ever attempted to share your life with him? Does he think so?

Of course, this kind of in-depth sharing shouldn't develop into a do-it-yourself psycho-analysis session over a plate of bacon and eggs. If you have to talk out serious problems, choose another time and place. The idea of this getting-to-know you business is that it should be fun, a positive time to get re-acquainted with the partner whom you thought you knew so well and a time that gives him a chance to realize all over again that you are a pretty fascinating person and that you are lucky to have each other.

If you listen (really listen) you will automatically become about 70 per cent more fascinating immediately. The rewards of actively listening to your husband are twofold. First, you will be astonished to find out what has happened to your man during the twenty years of more since you last paid attention. And, second, if you show so much interest in him, you will inevitably get his attention. He will want to know more about this woman, who has suddenly become such a brilliant conversationalist.

Now it's your turn. Communication must flow both ways and once you have captured his full attention (maybe for the first time in years) then you can finally talk to him. Share with him your inner thoughts and if you think you are doing all the work, taking all the initiative in revitalising your relationship, that cannot be a bad thing. If you don't remember, someone else may.

Yes, you may say, but I think this is the most artificial idea I have ever heard, what's more it seems somehow dis-honest. Does it? Does it seem artificial to look at the man you have been living with all those years and really see him? Does it seem artificial to work at re-creating the interest, and the love that you once had in your relationship? (And if you have never had these things in your marriage, isn't it time you did?)

The woman who considers this type of effort to be artificial is a woman we have met often in this book. She is the one who prefers to be totally natural and who insists (from God knows what subconscious compulsion) that the only really honest things in life are the ordinary things. What she means by that is the second rate things, the dull things. Some people think that 'real life' inevitably comes down to dental bills and new tyres for the car, but life consists of all the ways of living that there are, and every single one of them is real.

Revitalising a middle-aged marriage naturally takes some thought and effort, but then doesn't everything? Love is not a game for the lazy, the dull or the unimaginative, and any woman who worries about the 'honesty' of this kind of effort is usually the woman whose marriage has degenerated into a charade played by two strangers and I think any woman living with a man she doesn't even know is not only dishonest but downright degraded. Remember you can't have it both ways. You just cannot take the familiarity, the daily routine out of a middle-aged marriage without a bit of seemingly artificial effort. Of course it's going to seem 'put-on' at first, because it's a completely new way of looking at things, indeed a new attitude. It can't seem perfectly natural or comfortable if it's brand new, and good for that! Just what the doctor ordered.

But, never mind the doctor, here are some hints I suggest to help a middle-aged marriage out of the doldrums:

1. The Homebirds

As you know both husbands and wives contribute equally to the success of a marriage. An overly married couple will find as the years go by that they stay at home more and more. A certain amount of fatigue and boredom creeps in and each year seems to be 'too much trouble' to get out and about. This couple is usually glued to the television box night after night. They know more about Coronation Street and Starsky and Hutch than they do about each other. Weekends are usually spent pottering around the house and garden. How dull. No wonder they have little to say to each other, their marriage is drowning in boredom.

The 'homebirds' need to be jarred out of that rut and once again it's the woman who does not grow old who has to save the day. Why? you ask. Because first of all she is aware that there is a problem. Her husband knows that he's overtired (a sure sign of boredom) and gets increasingly depressed. Secondly, she's tuned into her life (and his) by a little thought and planning. And, thirdly, as we have noted so often before, women are the superior sex.

Of course, its easy for me to advise 'Pack up and go off for a weekend' or 'Dress up and go out to dinner' but these suggestions are expensive and most people will say 'We can't afford it.' Instead try some modest outings. A walk through the streets of a nearby town: anything to get you out of the rut.

One of the most helpful bits of advice I can give you is to remember that you don't necessarily have to go out at night. Today with women working, it's not always easy after a full day's work. Why not have lunch together, if it's only once a month.

One couple I know very often pack a Sunday lunch and go

for a drive taking the Sunday papers with them, not very exciting you may say, but at least it's different.

Another couple I know visit the local museum and art galleries in hopes of discovering something new.

There are many projects that a husband and wife can share. One couple I am friendly with, the wife told me the other day that her husband had discovered Admiral Nelson. 'Discovered Nelson' I asked, 'Yes,' she said. Through visiting the Naval Museum and reading letters from Lady Hamilton to Nelson he became interested in the man and read every book on the naval hero. His wife was so intrigued that she visited the museum and read the same books. Thus one sees another common interest. Each couple must work out the patterns of companionship that suits them best, and with a little imagination they can add a new dimension to their lives with such shared activities. The important thing, of course, is that they make a definite point to get out of those two well-worn ruts and into something new and different that they both enjoy. This is a wonderful, beautiful world and the possibilities are endless. And, what will grow from these shared interests? Many conversations and private jokes will be a renewed intimacy.

2. Independence

Shared activities are essential but too much togetherness can be just as bad for the middle-aged marriage as spending all the time apart. Psychologists are always telling us that it is quality and not quantity of the time spent together that counts.

The idea of togetherness has been so over-blown by the media that many couples think they must spend every single moment together but ultimately this stifling togetherness can be devastating to any relationship.

Of course, shared activities and interests certainly are important to any marriage but there must be an understanding and willingness to allow the other person an individual life of his or her own. No married person can stay happy as one half of a Siamese twin so please don't overdo the togetherness. Don't make a religion of it. Having an opportunity to pursue one's own interest is so important because a degree of individuality helps to get one out of that middle-aged rut and makes one a more interesting person.

Having an independent interest also creates a little mystery, a sense of the unknown in even the most long-lived relationship and each partner will retain a sense of identity. The key word is balance. Each couple must strike some sensible degree of balance between the shared time and interests that mean companionship and another of private interests that permit a healthy degree of individuality. We all need moments alone to reinforce our individual uniqueness, to feel free, to think, to experiment and yes, even to dream.

Unfortunately, women are often the worst offenders in the destruction of individual privacy. What are you doing? Where are you going? What time will you be back? Treating a husband like a child. So you see it is healthy to rethink your attitude towards privacy. Every adult needs some quiet time alone.

3. Grandparents

I couldn't finish this chapter without mentioning grandparents. Grandchildren are wonderful, someone once said, 'It's all fun being a grandparent, it's like having children without any of the headaches,' but some couples become what I would call the 'Professional Grandparents', the ones who put their own marriage into mothballs. Couples, whose every leisure hour is spent with their grandchildren, are the couples who have not readjusted their lives to reality and are playing at Mama Bear, Papa Bear and Baby Bear. They are the couple who want to take over their children and their children's children. Remember your children have a right to their children. The over-indulgent grandparents should analyse the time spent with their grandchildren and cut it in half, then they should concentrate on rebuilding that just-the-two-of-us relationship.

CHAPTER IX

PLASTIC SURGERY — IS IT FOR YOU?

I am sure every woman over forty has done it. You have probably done it too. When you are putting on your make-up, combing your hair or dressing for an important occasion. You look at yourself in the mirror, place your fingers at the side of your face and pull up. Instantly you look younger, more rested and happier. Wouldn't it be exciting to give your face (as well as your morale) that permanent lift? Plastic Surgery can do it but, do you dare?

Why not? The face lift, once the exclusive prerogative of film stars and members of the jet set, is now becoming commonplace. As a result, the number of men and women having plastic surgery has increased phenomenally and not only are these patients from a different income bracket but their attitude is totally different. In the past, people tended to be very secretive about plastic surgery, but not any more.

What would be the best age for having a face lift?

This has always been a leading question, since cosmetic surgery creates a unique medical situation. It is the only operation that you tell the doctor when you need it; not vice versa.

So how will you decide? Apart from the psychological and financial side the answer is 'Sooner the Better'. At least that seems to be the attitude of leading surgeons. I think the age when you should be thinking of face lifts is between forty and fifty five. Important as age is, many surgeons consider the over-all physical condition to be another prime factor. The person who is healthy and who hasn't over-indulged in food or drink will have the best results. Some surgeons urge their patients to go into training a few months before surgery, on a regimen that makes alcohol, coffee and even tea a big 'NO'. They also prescribe a high protein diet with lots of Vitamin A foods.

A lot of people I know have had minor corrective surgery. At the first sign of a drooping eyelid or pouchy jaw, the patient undergoes this corrective surgery, which has several advantages:

1. Compared to a complete face lift, it is less traumatic to the tissue.
2. The results are so subtle that there is never any need to explain how you have managed to put back the clock.
3. It virtually prevents the face from ever looking old.

This approach may not be for you, but it is definitely the thing of the future. Young people today will more than likely live their middle years in an atmosphere that treats a visit to the plastic surgeon as casually as a visit to the dentist.

What about Scars?
Well that depends on what you have done. In the standard face lift, the hair is parted just beyond the hairline at the temple and an incision is made, it continues, within the hairline, down towards the ear and this scar is completely hidden. If the operation includes an eye lift, the

scars are hidden in the natural folds above the eyelid. If an eyebrow lift is needed, the suture line is concealed first within the upper hairline of the brow. If a double chin is the problem, an incision is made just under the chin line.

What is the Cost?

There is no such thing in plastic surgery as a standard fee. When you realise that your face lift may include one or any combination of the operations I have described, it's easy to see why surgeons are wary about quoting prices to the general public. However, it is possible to get a general estimate of the cost and most people are surprised to find that the dream of a face lift is well within their financial means.

Natural approach to rejuvenating the face.

I am quite sure by now that some of my readers are asking, 'Is there a non-medical approach to lifting and rejuvenating my face?' The exciting answer is, '**YES**'.

There are several things you can do — simple, inexpensive and safe techniques — which will make your face appear lifted, younger and vital. I am always surprised when I give lectures that these techniques are unknown to so many women. They are all easy, inexpensive and readily available.

The Beauty Legend

In France, in the seventeenth century, a courtesan named Ninar de Lenclos became a legend in her time, not only because, in her later years, she retained her youthful appearance to a startling degree, but it has been said that young men fell madly in love with her when she was well past seventy years old. Of course that may or may not appeal to you, but it would be fun in the future to have the chance to say no.

Mystery and legend surround the means she used to retain her beauty, but one of her secrets is said to have been a series of facial exercises that kept her skin elastic and firm and lifted her facial contours in a perpetually youthful manner.

Although the actual techniques she used are lost in the mists of time, some very contemporary beauties are using modern facial exercises and getting age-defying results.

How do they work?

They work on exactly the same principle that body exercises work. When you stop to think about it, the face is composed of bones, muscles and nerves, just as the body is. If the facial muscles are kept toned and firm, then the face will retain its youthful contours. The skin will be firm because it is supported by the solid muscle underneath, and the skin will have improved colour and texture and elasticity. Why? Because any exercise, whether it's for the face or body, not only tones the muscles but improves the circulation which feeds the cells and helps with the disposal of wastes. This is why facial exercises, consistently practised, bring such satisfying results, lifting facial contours and at the same time minimising wrinkles.

Yes, facial exercises do work, and remember they only work if you keep at it. Unfortunately, most people do them for a week or so and then stop. These are some of the most effective facial exercises:

To lift a Sagging Jowl

Pull the left mouth corner to the left as far as you can, at the same time, raise your eyebrows. Keeping the mouth pulled to the side, slowly wink the left eye. Now tightly squint the left eye and wrinkle your nose. Hold for a moment and slowly release the muscle tension. (Repeat all the exercises with the right side of the face).

Now this may sound utterly mad and somewhat weird but it works. Do this each day and after a month you will see some readily visible result. Facial exercises will work as long as you do.

Forehead Lines

Horizontal lines on the forehead are one of the most common forms of wrinkles. Many women appear to have corrugated foreheads instead of the smooth, serene brows associated with feminine beauty. What is more, plastic surgery won't remove these lines, but why not get rid of them yourself?

Forehead lines are never the result of age, but only of faulty facial habits. The solution — apply three horizontal strips of masking tape to your relaxed forehead whenever you are at home alone. The tape will tell you when your forehead wrinkles. You will be surprised how often you are raising (or trying to raise) your eyebrows. Some women only do this when they are talking. Think when the phone rings you say, 'Hello' and the eyebrows shoot up toward the hairline. Others find that the forehead is a constant accompaniment to their thoughts.

Whatever the degree of your problem, the old masking tape will pay a double dividend. Not only will you break yourself of this unattractive facial habit, but your forehead will remain smooth and unlined for several hours after the very first tape application.

The tendency to pull the mouth to one side is another wrinkle-making facial habit that can be corrected with tape. Relax your face and apply the tape from the corner of your mouth to the side of your nose, starting at the mouth and gently pulling the tape up as you apply it. You may apply the tape to just one side or both sides depending on your particular facial habit.

Snap

The techniques I have mentioned so far work but it takes time, so how would you like to have an instant face lift? One simple gadget can give you a 'mini-lift? I am talking about an elastic headband. It will lift years from your face (you would be surprised how many famous beauties would not leave their homes without one of these painless, do-it-yourself face lifters). The headband is just that. Slide it up over your face and above the hairline. The band pulls the hair up and gently lifts your facial contours in the process.

After you are through gazing at yourself in pleasant amazement you can arrange your hair over the headband or cover the band with a scarf. I kid you not, you will drop ten years in the time it takes to put on one of these headbands. Is it comfortable? Yes, as long as it is correctly applied; pure hell if you don't get it just right. So practise.

Where can I buy one?

There are several good headbands on the markets. Many beauty salons and sports shops sell them and often they are advertised in magazines.

Well what do you think now about improving your face whether by plastic surgery or the natural way? In one of my recent lectures one lady said to me, 'I'd rather stick with what I've got.' My answer to that is: 'While the rest of the world is improving why let your body and face fall apart?' I would think that any woman wants to look her best at all times.

If you are worried about the opinions of your acquaintances and co-workers, you are in for a shock. Most people are not as interested in us as we would like to think. They are totally involved in their own lives their own problems and actually give us very little thought. What is more, our relationships with the people on the periphery of our lives can change without warning. For instance, one of my patients told me she wanted to improve her looks. I advised her, as I have in this book, on diet and natural beauty aids and facial exercises but one of the girls in her office had told her to stay as she was, so she almost gave up on the idea of improving herself. Then one day she said to me, 'But what about my husband? He also said, 'Don't bother, you look fine to me'. Then she turned to me and said, 'But I don't need a new face for him, it's for myself.' Today she looks entirely different, far more radiant and youthful looking. When I asked her recently what her husband thought she said he was very pleased and enjoyed going out with this more attractive woman.

But remember the most important person to please is yourself. That is the ultimate answer to 'what will people say?'

CHAPTER X

A STATE OF MIND

In this book we have met many women who are ageless and we have met many who can't be bothered. The differences between them seem innumerable at first but, actually, there is only one difference and that is attitude. In every case the woman who can't be bothered is victimised by a state of mind: a rigid, ingrained mental state that confines her to a limited, stagnating and negative, old way of life.

Many philosophers, scientists and religious teachers have clearly demonstrated that by changing negative attitudes and replacing them with positive viewpoints, the woman, who 'can't be bothered' could change her entire way of life, her physical health and even the rate at which she ages.

Will she ever change? I wouldn't like to bet on it. Her state of mind has become ingrained. But, if I were to bet I would put my money on you, because if you have read this far you have clearly proved that your attitudes are not set in concrete, that you already have many positive outlooks necessary for growth and change and that you can become the winner and not grow old.

Let us talk about the vital importance of attitude or call it spirit if you like. We have discussed health, style, exercise and many many other things, so let us see how attitudes can create or destroy and how they can prevent you from becoming old.

A Scientific Reality

Experiments have proven that the body mechanisms respond to mental attitudes. Often when patients are given a placebo, a harmless sugar pill, they think it will make them well. Many doctors, who are even sceptical about the power of the mind over the body, still use placebos in their daily practice. We are all familiar with the power of hypnotic suggestion. There have been many instances of hypnotised subjects who experienced an extreme physical reaction to a mental suggestion.

There have also been many recorded examples of the destructive power that the mind can exert on the body. In primitive societies the witch-doctor can often kill by suggestion. Through ritual, myth and magic that is accepted by the entire primitive society, the witch-doctor convinces the victim that he is doomed and at the appointed moment he just lies down and dies.

We too, of course have our rituals, myths and magic and our tribal convictions.

Think of the ritual litany of the women who can't be bothered, 'When I was younger I used to . . .'; 'When we get older we slow down'; 'No fool like an old fool'; 'Oh! it would be ridiculous at my age' and 'Why can't she grow old gracefully?' and so on to her very last day, which such negative destructive thoughts will certainly hasten.

On the other hand a positive dynamic attitude will stimulate the mind and keep the body young. The rejuvenating effect of mind has been observed by people of many ages. Many doctors and scientists are deeply aware of the relationship between ageing and mental attitude.

Mental Attitude

The influence of the mind on the body has been noted by every religion and philosophy since this world began. The Bible tells us 'Be ye transformed by the renewing of the mind' and 'As a man thinketh in his heart, so is he.' Charles Tillmore is one of the many contemporary philosophers who stressed the importance of attitude in combating old age. When he was fifty he wrote, 'About three years ago the belief in old age began to take hold of me. I began to get wrinkled and grey, my knees tottered and a great weakness came over me. I did not discern the cause at once, but I found in my dreams I was associating with old people, and it gradually dawned on me that I was coming into this phase of race belief.

'I spent hours and hours silently affirming my unity with the infinite energy of the one true God. I associated with the young, danced with them, sang with them.'

At ninety-three Charles Tillmore was still demonstrating the power of attitude over age. He was still at his desk daily, still actively involved with the world around him. The power of the mind is enormous and this is why I am in favour of colouring grey hair, having your face lifted if it needs it, exercising to keep your body slim and lithe, dressing in contemporary fashions, keeping your mind actively engrossed in the present and the future. All of these things will help your mind combat the idea of old age and prove to you that you need not get old.

The Secret of Youth

Throughout the world there are rejuvenators, mystery medical magicians who keep the great and glamorous in the prime of life, never mind what the calendar may say. These doctors can be theorists, but one thing is certain, they have to be realists, because their success or failure is so obvious in the mirrors of their patients. No scientific jargon will con an ageing beauty when her mirror clearly proves that her doctor has failed. All these rejuvenators have one thing in common that contributes to their success — they work to build positive attitudes in the minds of their patients.

Upon becoming a widow a woman often feels that her active life has ended. This mental attitude is demonstrated by her general lack of interest and ageing appearance. On the other hand some widows take on a new lease of life — they embark on a new job, find fresh interests and adopt a positive attitude which has a rejuvenating effect and also improves their appearance.

But Hutchnecher also noted that other widows actually blossom. They may enter into competition for a new husband, start a new career, find new interests and such women, with a positive attitude toward their life actually tend to change their age for the better. Positive attitudes do have a rejuventating effect on the body and you needn't age.

You must ruthlessly reject all those negative, limiting, age-making opinions of the woman who can't be bothered. If you can't escape such a woman, at least train yourself to tune her out and more importantly, develop a rebellious attitude to her negative 'vibes'.

Of course the knowledge that thought has the power to influence our bodies is not new, even though scientists are only now beginning to recognise this influence. Spiritual leaders of all creeds as well as metaphysicians have known this truth for centuries.

What is your Age?

Never answer that question, if you can help it. Of course you have to, at the passport office, to traffic policemen and at the personnel departments. But, once you have dealt with these unavoidable snoops, keep your age to yourself. There is a very good reason for this advice and it has nothing to do with vanity.

If you agree with me that the condition of your body is directly related to your mental image, you can see that telling your true age will only create needless obstacles. If you constantly mention the passing years, then you are setting in motion the destructive mental forces that will remind your body of age. And dwelling on your age will also influence the attitudes of people around you.

If you tell your age, if you discuss your age, other people immediately form a whole series of impressions and con-clusions about you, based on their concept of a person in your age bracket. They will immediately categorise you and their concept of forty plus, which may be negative and limited, becomes the basis of their relationship with you.

I have told you, you are not getting older, you are getting better. You also know that woman in this modern world, with longer life spans and greater opportunities, makes you the youngest forty, fifty or sixty year old this world has ever known. As you realise there is no need to grow old, you will reflect this truth: that age is not an absolute, it is relative.

If age were an absolute, like a chemical reaction or a mathematical equation, then we would all age at exactly the same rate. But, a quick glance at the women around you will prove that age is a concept not a reality.

The woman who does not look her age is literally able to rise above those who do, both physically and mentally.

So whenever it is possible, keep your age to yourself. Not because you are being coy and not because you are trying to be what you are not (I don't know of anyone who would want to be twenty or thirty again) but because you refuse to be limited by the negative, conventional attitudes that most people have towards middle age.

Banish for ever any stereotypes you may be harbouring regarding the life style, the abilities and appearance of various ages. Look past forty and fifty for a moment: what is the popular concept of a woman of eighty? What is it we see? A deal little old lady, a shawl around her shoulders, a bundle of knitting in her lap. Oh! yes, she is sweet, dull and a bit simple. But, let us now look at some women whose attitudes have freed them from these stereotypes.

Marlene Dietrich — eighty or almost (unbelievable isn't it, with the figure and looks of a young girl). Barbara Cartland — let us say late seventies. What a dynamic character, full of vitality and the looks of a woman half her age.

Think of the number of famous women from late fifties upwards whose looks and figures defy their years and I am convinced they are as they are through positive thinking.

What do you get out of life?

I have found after giving lectures for years and seeing patients every day, that most women feel they must make sacrifices; very often these women have been so beaten down in life that they don't demand enough from it, from themselves or from those around them.

I always think how sad it is when so many women become servants in their own homes. They allow themselves to deteriorate so that they can't be inspiring as a mother or desirable as a wife. They have so often allowed their families to restrict their personal growth. This should never be tolerated.

If anyone reading this book has become a servant to her family, then its time she handed in her notice. The situation can be changed and should be. It's good for you, your husband and it is essential for your children. Psychologists will agree that the most valuable gift anyone can give their children is to demonstrate to them that being an adult has privileges and advantages, and that is what they can look forward to, because it offers many rewards. Young people must be made to see that as the old army saying goes 'Rank has privileges.'

But, in this country today, sadly, the adults have abdicated and let their children rule. It is no wonder that many young people treat older people with contempt — they are entitled to because we have betrayed them. All too often we have presented them with a terrible picture of middle age — a grey, dreary, negative and depressing time of life typified by middle age spread, dentures and grey hair. What is their future? They know only too well that the calendar is leading them on to their own middle age and if they despairingly reject that gloomy, negative future who can blame them if they sweepingly reject the customs, manners and morals of the adult world.

So becoming ageless is not just a vanity kick. The woman who has made up her mind not to get old can demonstrate to her children and to young people around her that life is wonderful and this world really is beautiful, that the mature years ahead can be a time of excitement, creativity and fulfilment She can, by example, instil into her children those positive attitudes that will allow them to look forward to maturity with optimism and anticipation and, believe me, young people today need their heroines.

Please don't misunderstand me, I am not suggesting that you once again martyr yourself for your family, this time by trying to look young for the sake of the children. No, look young and ageless for yourself. Become self-confident, an individual who radiates independence, with your own ideas and interests, who has the courage to let her personality shine.

Why grow old? Surely I have proved in this book that you need not. Develop your mind and have an inner rewarding life. Stop thinking of yourself as 'The Better Half' or 'Just a Housewife' and don't worry about the effect on your family or your friends, or society in general. It will be wonderful, because a woman who refuses to grow old is an inspiration to everyone and that is just what this world needs.